HEALTHY CHOICES

AVOIDING HARMFUL SUBSTANCES

Cath Senker

PowerKiDS
press.
New York

Published in 2008 by The Rosen Publishing Group, Inc.
29 East 21st Street, New York, NY 10010

First Edition

Consultant: Jayne Wright
Design: Sarah Borny

The publishers would like to thank the following for allowing
us to reproduce their pictures in this book:
Corbis; 6, 8, 11, 12 / Hodder Wayland Picture Library; 7, 9, 14
15, 16, 17, 19, 20, 21 / Zul Mukhida 4, 5, 13, 18

Library of Congress Cataloging-in-Publication Data

Senker, Cath.
  Avoiding harmful substances / Cath Senker. — 1st ed.
     p. cm. — (Healthy choices)
  Includes index.
  ISBN 978-1-4042-4304-0 (library binding)
  1. Drugs—Juvenile literature. 2. Toxicology—Juvenile literature. I. Title.
  RM301.17.S46 2008
  615'.1—dc22
                                        2007032803

Manufactured in China

Contents

What are drugs?

 A drug is something that changes the way your body works. It makes you feel different.

Medicines are drugs that can make you better if you are sick. They can kill germs and stop a pain from hurting. Medicines can stop you from getting nasty diseases.

It is important to choose the right kind of medicine.

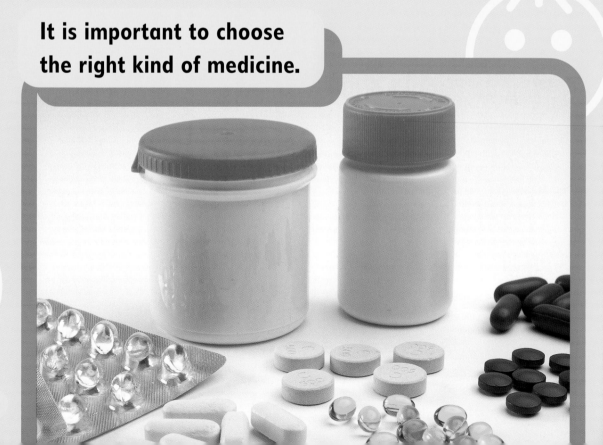

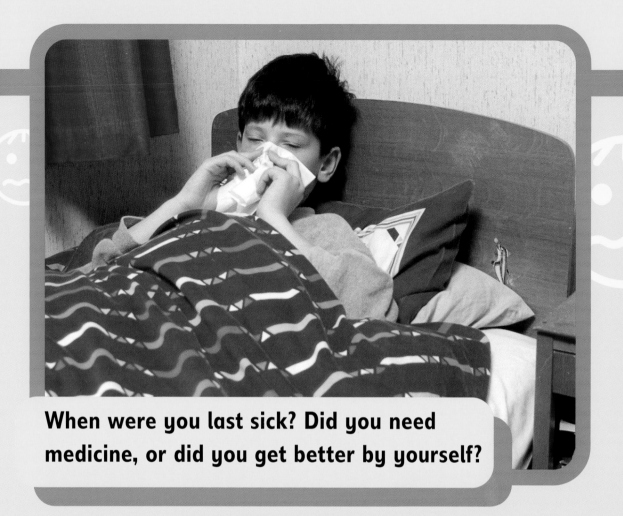

When were you last sick? Did you need medicine, or did you get better by yourself?

If you take the wrong drug, or you take too much, it can harm you. You might get sleepy or sick to your stomach, or get a rash.

Alcohol and cigarettes are also drugs. They can make people sick. Some people use powerful drugs that are against the law. They can be very dangerous, too.

I feel sick. What can I do?

 We all get colds, sore throats, and stomachaches. Usually, your body gets better all by itself.

Do you need a drug for a bug? Sometimes you need some medicine to help you get better. There are no cures for colds and the flu, but medicine can make you feel more comfortable.

An adult

can buy you

medicines for

coughs and

colds, and aches

and pains. They

can be bought from a

drugstore or a supermarket.

The package tells you the **dose** you should take. Soon

you will feel well again.

Where should medicines be kept at home?

(Answer on page 23)

Why do I need to take medicine?

 Feeling sick and need a pill? Sometimes you have something wrong with you that won't get better by itself. Maybe the person looking after you doesn't know what is making you sick.

If you're really sick, go to the doctor quick! The doctor will see what is wrong. You might need a special medicine. The doctor will write a note called a **prescription**. An adult will take it to the drugstore to get the right medicine.

Medicines can come as liquids, pills, and creams. Some are injected or sniffed up the nose.

Use your medicine just as the doctor says. Too little and you won't get better. Too much and you might get more sick.

Why should you never take a medicine that is for someone else?

(Answer on page 23)

What are herbal medecines?

 Not all medicines come from the doctor. Some people go to health food stores. They can buy medicines made from herbs and other plants. People should be careful with them, just like with all medicines.

To get advice, you can go to see a herbalist. The *herbalist* knows about using herbs as medicines. People may choose to visit a *homeopath*. Homeopaths use different kinds of medicines from the ones doctors use.

Do you know anyone who uses herbal or homeopathic medicines? Have you used them yourself, and did they help?

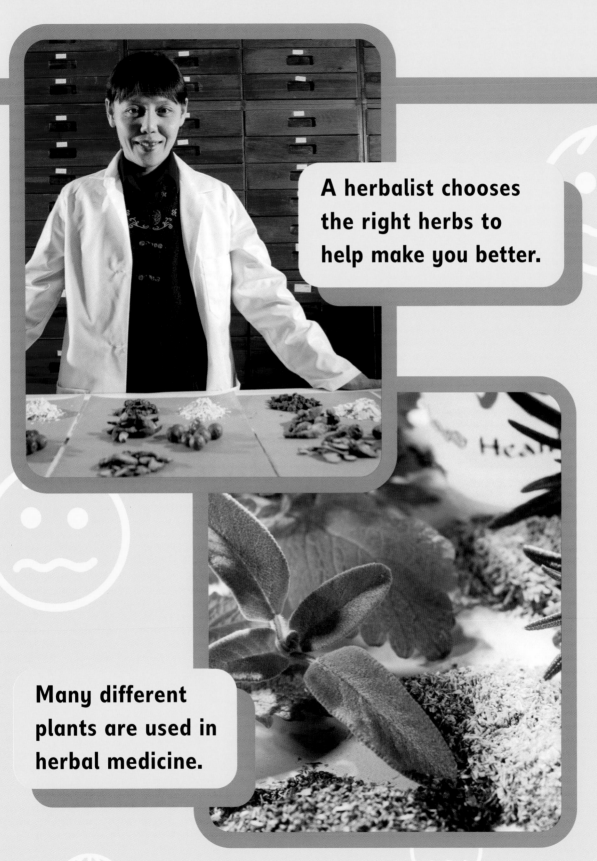

A herbalist chooses the right herbs to help make you better.

Many different plants are used in herbal medicine.

Why do I need shots?

When you were little, you probably had some shots.

What have you had shots for?
(Answer on page 23)

The doctor uses a small needle that goes under your skin. This tiny little pinprick can stop you from getting sick.

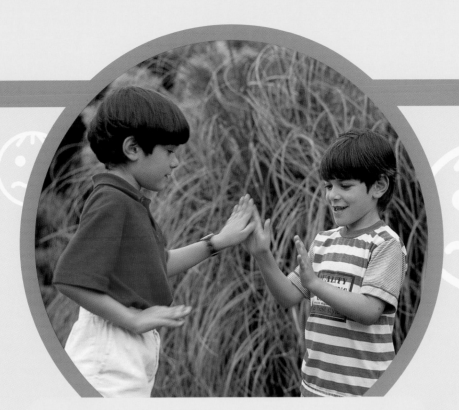

Shots help to stop you catching diseases and keep you healthy.

The needle contains a drug. It can protect you from nasty diseases, such as **measles**, **mumps,** and **TB**. It works like this. The measles drug contains a very weak kind of measles. Your body kills the measles easily. If you're ever close to people with the real disease, your body already knows how to fight it off.

Why does my friend have an inhaler?

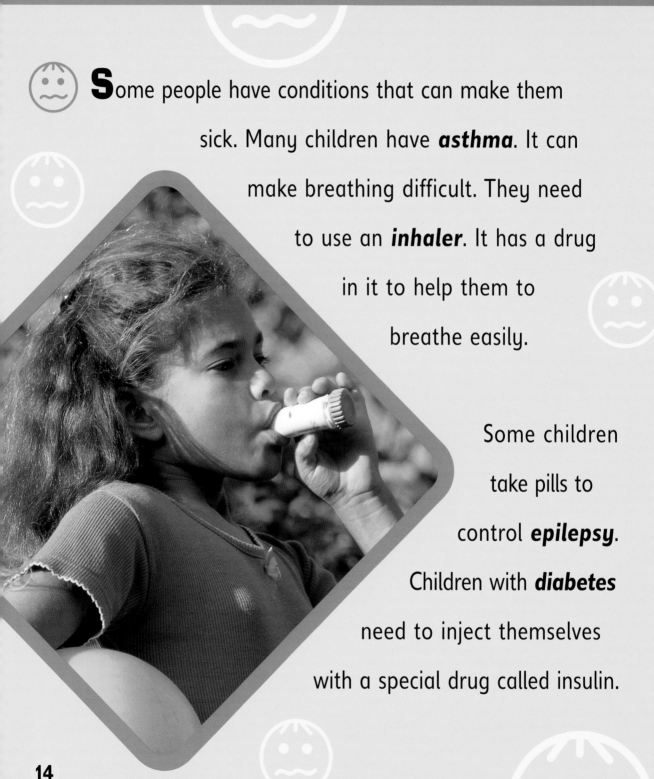

Some people have conditions that can make them sick. Many children have **asthma**. It can make breathing difficult. They need to use an **inhaler**. It has a drug in it to help them to breathe easily.

Some children take pills to control **epilepsy**. Children with **diabetes** need to inject themselves with a special drug called insulin.

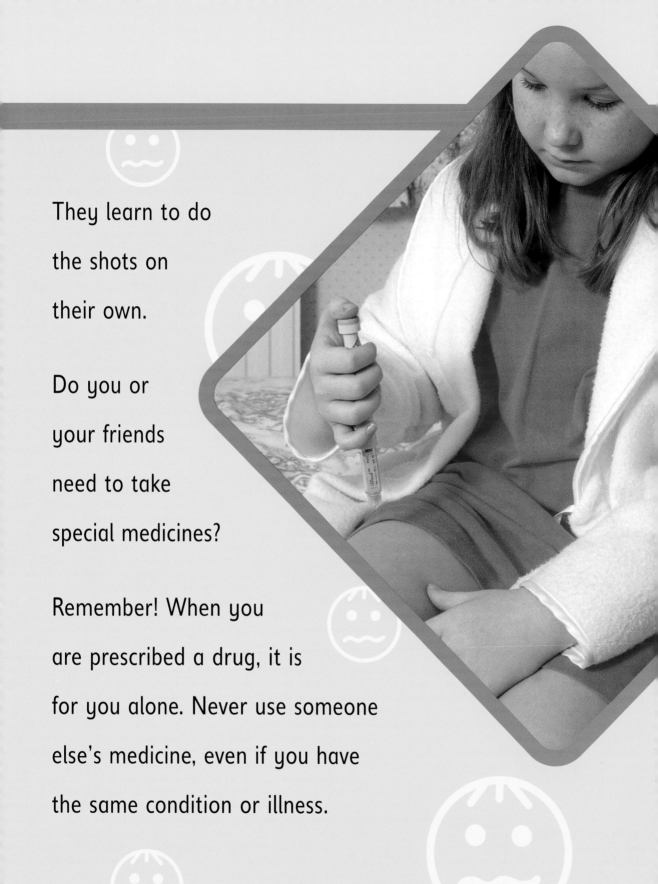

They learn to do
the shots on
their own.

Do you or
your friends
need to take
special medicines?

Remember! When you
are prescribed a drug, it is
for you alone. Never use someone
else's medicine, even if you have
the same condition or illness.

What are household chemicals for?

 Household chemicals do a useful job. Cleaning fluids are needed to make your home clean and fresh. Have you ever broken a favorite toy? An adult probably used strong glue to fix it.

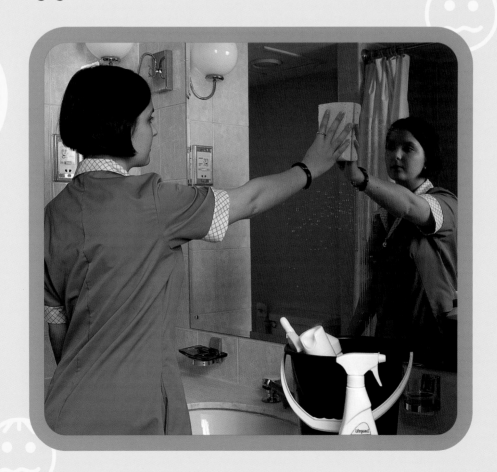

This symbol is on dangerous chemicals, so that you know they could be harmful.

Household chemicals are very powerful. They can harm you if you don't use them in the right way. Strong cleaners such as bleach could make you very sick if you swallowed them by accident. Some kinds of glue have a strong smell. It makes you feel very unwell.

Which household chemicals do you have at home? Learn to keep away from them. Look after yourself— leave chemicals on the shelf!

Why do people drink alcohol?

 Many adults drink alcohol, because it helps them to feel more lively or relaxed.

Alcohol is a powerful drug. People should think before they drink. If they drink too much, they will get drunk. Drunk people can be noisy and frightening. They may not 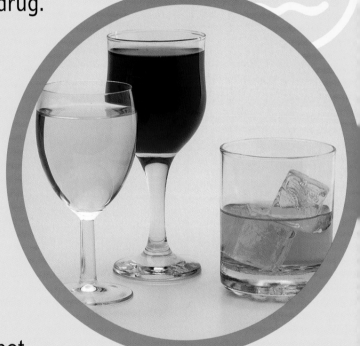 know what they are doing. They can cause accidents.

Do you know which drinks have alcohol in them?

(Answer on page 23)

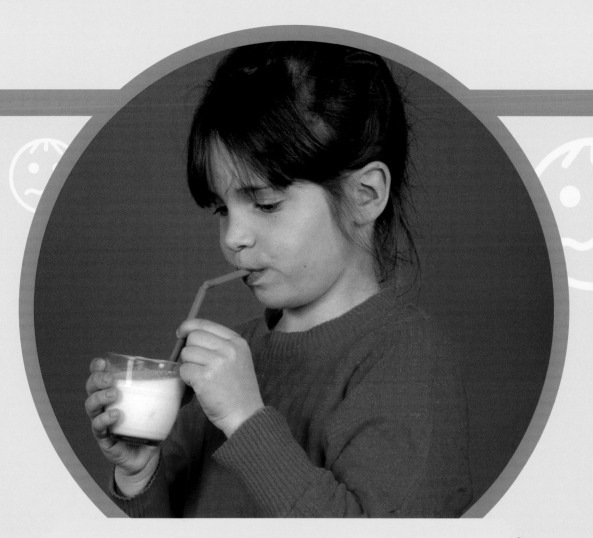

Go for healthy drinks such as milk and juice. This girl is enjoying a delicious milkshake.

Alcohol is too strong for children's small bodies. It can make them drunk very quickly. Some alcoholic drinks have fruit in them and look like they are for children. Beware—these drinks could be harmful.

Why is smoking so bad for you?

 Many people smoke. They say it helps them to relax and feel good.

But smoking makes people smell—and their clothes, too. It makes them sick. The chemicals in cigarette smoke are poisonous. They go into the smoker's body and damage the lungs. It can then become hard for them to breathe.

What would you do if someone offered you a cigarette?

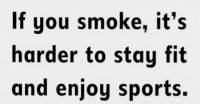

If you smoke, it's harder to stay fit and enjoy sports.

Smoking makes people's bodies need more cigarettes. They become *addicted*. They find it hard to stop smoking, even if they want to. It's better not to start smoking in the first place.

If people around you smoke, you breathe in the dangerous chemicals, too. This is bad for your health.

Glossary and index

measles 13   A disease that gives you a fever and small red spots all over your body.

mumps 13   A disease that makes the sides of your face swell up.

prescription 8   A piece of paper on which the doctor writes down the medicine you need.

TB (Tuberculosis) 13   A serious disease that causes swellings on the lungs and other parts of the body.

Answers to questions:

P.7   Medicines should be kept in a locked cabinet, out of the reach of children.

P.9   If you take a medicine that is for someone else, it could be dangerous for you. All people are different and the medicines they need are often different, too.

P.12   Children in the United States usually have shots for diphtheria, tetanus, whooping cough, polio, meningitis, measles, mumps, and rubella.

P.18   These are some drinks that have alcohol in them: beer, wine, whisky, vodka, gin.

Finding out more

Books to read:

Avoiding Drugs

by Patricia J. Murphy (Lerner Publications, 2005)

Drugs (What About Health?)

by Fiona Waters (Hodder Wayland, 2004)

Let's Talk About Alcohol

by Sarah Levete (Stargazer Books, 2007)

Let's Talk About Drugs

by Sarah Levete (Stargazer Books, 2007)

The Nosmo King

by Phyllis Abbott (Yvonne Hedley, 1996)

Web Sites

Due to the changing nature of Internet links, PowerKids Press has developed an online list of Web sites related to the subject of this book. This site is regularly updated. Please use this link to access this list:

www.powerkidslinks.com/health/avoid

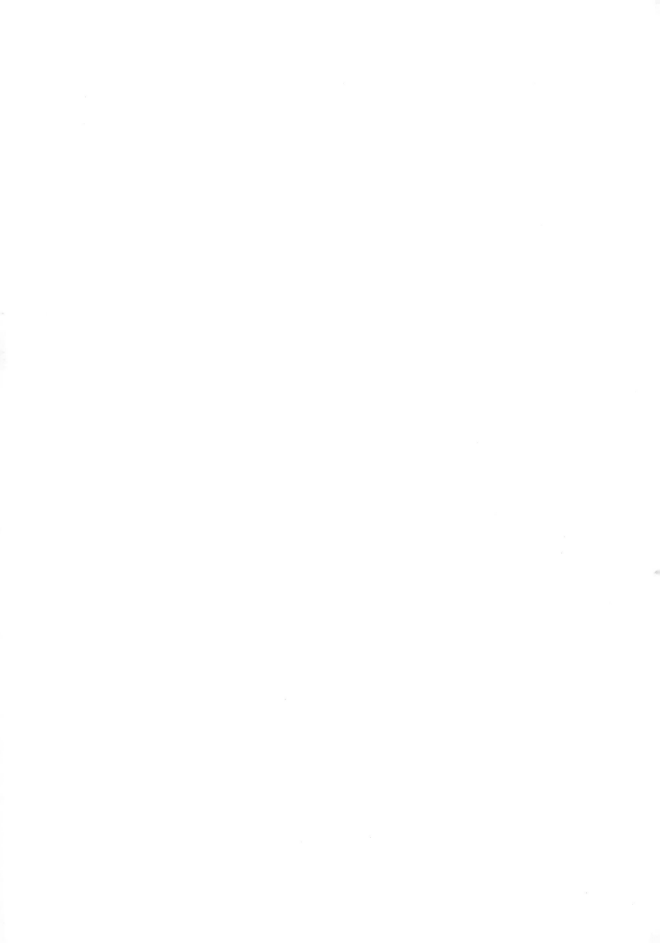